MY PATH TO HEAVEN ON EARTH

LOSING LIFE AS I KNEW IT AND FINDING H.O.P.E.

BILL CLARKE

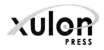

Fred and Rosemarie,

May God bless you on
this wild ride we call life
and may you find your path
to heaven on earth.

Paul Clarke

Table of Contents

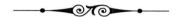

Introduction

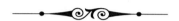

I never thought I would be writing a book. From a very young age, I had my life planned. I was going to be a rich businessman. When I was just ten years old, I opened my first business, making homemade root beer and selling it to the neighborhood kids. I got a lucky break at age thirteen when I was hired to work at a local hardware store. I fell in love with retail and immediately set my sights on owning my own hardware business one day.

After college, I went to work as an assistant manager at a local grocery chain. I progressed quickly to a corporate position. I eventually became the director of a large chain. Over the years, I worked hard and earned a position as a vice president. That led to more jobs with various retail chains and a big salary. We owned two homes, put three kids through college and traveled extensively.

Life was good.

However, my comfortable life took a drastic turn when I suffered a severe stroke at the age of 55 in

2005. The stroke robbed me of my executive-level brain function, but left me with an amazing gift. A switch was flipped in my brain, which opened my mind to a new philosophical and spiritual way of thinking.

This is an account of my journey from living large, as a successful businessman, through my life-changing stroke and struggle to create a new "normal."

If you believe in God, but wonder why bad things happen to good people, or you are currently facing severe hardship, then you may gain insight from my experience. I've come to the conclusion that God's will be done. We can't change that, but we do have a choice. We can either be dragged along on our life journey, kicking and screaming, or we can accept his will, trust in Him and enjoy the ride.

CHAPTER ONE

Life Before My Stroke

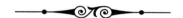

I was born in 1950, the second of ten in small town Ohio into a middle class family. My mother, her two brothers, and mother and father, a Jewish family, survived the Nazis by immigrating to the United States. Her grandparents were not so lucky. Wilhelm and Emilia were deported and executed in the Maly Trosinec death camp. My dad drove a DUCK (amphibian truck) during D-Day on Omaha beach. He told me the shore was heavily mined. When a landing craft hit a mine it.exploded and all were killed. He spoke of his craft landing safely in shallow water, and he wading passed body after body in a sea of red. With the extreme challenges to survive that my parents faced; It's a miracle that I was ever born. Yet somehow God was looking after me even before I was born. I am sure he has a plan for my life. I plan to find it.

Because of my loving parents and nine high-energy siblings, I had a fun-filled childhood. Our days were filled with games we made up, chores, swimming or sledding and sports of every kind. I was a natural leader and quickly learned that playing army was my favorite game... I could make myself the general, and all the younger kids would willingly follow my orders. Thanks to the education that mom and dad gave me at home, I excelled in school and earned a Bachelor of Science degree in management. I didn't earn my foundation in life, but I worked hard and made the best of what was given to me. I was blessed with intelligence. My parents instilled values, a strong work ethic and an appreciation for the Catholic faith in me.There was nothing I did to get this great start in life nor is there anything any of us can do to control our birth circumstances. I now realize how blessed I was. Looking back, my idyllic childhood was just the first evidence of God's love for me. Thanks to my experience in hardware I landed a job in the sporting goods department in the city. One day, while checking out the binocular inventory I spotted a new female in shoes. So, God gave me my bride to be, right where he knew I would find her while I was goofing off at work. We dated about a year. Somehow we both knew we were meant for each other and got married right after I finished college. God blessed us with two daughters and a son, and later nine grandchildren.

Life had treated me kindly. My health was good, and my family's future was nothing but optimistic. Little did I know, life as I knew it was about to change.

CHAPTER TWO

The Stroke

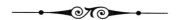

The weather was terrible in Augusta, Georgia, on January 29, 2005. Temperatures were at freezing, and we were getting a snow/sleet mix; very unusual for this southern city.

I'd just finished a store visit for the national drug store chain where I worked as the district manager. My normal routine was to make a quick stop for a cup of coffee mid- morning. I would take this time to review my notes from the last store visit and prepare for the next one. That day I went for a milkshake, instead of coffee; unusual for health-conscious me.

The day before had been grueling for my team. I spent all day loading and unload boxes of pharmacy files and product with my crew at the drug chain. We moved everything from the old Clearwater store to the new one. I didn't have to help, but that was my leadership style. I believed in doing the dirty work, right along with my team. I was a regular on the tennis and basketball courts, so the severe neck and shoulder pain I experienced that night came as a surprise. As I sipped my shake the next day, I was thankful that the pain in my neck from the previous night had subsided.

As I finished the shake, I picked up my backpack and started toward the exit. Suddenly, my backpack felt incredibly heavy. Something seemed to be pulling me down as I tried to leave the restaurant. Fortunately, an alert employee noticed my struggle and asked if I was okay. I understood, but could only shake my head *no*. Then he or she (I don't remember) asked if they should call 911. This time I nodded. *Yes! Yes!* I didn't realize it yet, but I had suffered a severe stroke and was paralyzed on my left side. It was the weight of my own body that was dragging me down. At the time, my brain was too wounded to understand anything. Still, I knew something was terribly wrong.

The next thing I remember is waking up on the floor, dazed and confused. The EMT asked if he could call my next of kin. I managed to give him my cell phone and my wife's name.

The ride to the hospital was wild, with the speed of the ambulance and the siren blaring; yet, it was comforting. The EMT sat beside me, assuring me that he had everything under control. Doctors were waiting at University Hospital, just a little farther down the street. His reassurances calmed me, and I wasn't afraid.

The EMT suspected a stroke, and he knew every minute counted. Fortunately, the nearby University Hospital had a stroke ward with the TPA drug (like drain cleaner for blocked arteries); but it had to be administered quickly.

In retrospect, I know God was watching over me. I happened to stay in town that day because of the driving conditions. Had I been in one of my country stores, I would never have gotten the TPA drug in time for my miraculous recovery. If I'd been driving when I had the stroke, I could have been killed and perhaps taken someone else with me. To some, it might seem like a random series of fortunate coincidences. However, I think coincidence is God's way of remaining anonymous; and there has been plenty of that in my life before, during and after my stroke.

Events that followed are a blur to me. I recall a doctor asking me questions about the current date, where I was and who the president was. I remember repeating that I was at McDonald's. I thought I was still there, since it was the last thing I remembered. After that my world became a jumble of noises. I don't know if I was conscious or unconscious at the time.

At one point I remember thinking, "What's that knocking sound?" I heard it, over and over. It was so irritating. Then someone told me to hold my leg still. I now know that I was being administered TPA through my leg while I was in the MRI machine. Next, a doctor stood over me asking me to sign a document for permission to operate on my brain. (I still can't believe they ask that of someone who is obviously incapable of making such a decision!)

I signed the document, but fortunately, brain surgery was unnecessary. The TPA worked; the bleeding from the hemorrhage stopped.

My next vivid memory is of my wife, Donna, and my children by my bedside in the ICU. I couldn't comprehend what was happening and wondered why they were there. I learned that I was paralyzed on my left side and couldn't talk. I remember feeling vulnerable and helpless, but Donna was there to comfort me. What a special gal I chose for my wife thirty-three years and three kids ago. Donna has been an angel and further evidence of God in my life. She was by my side caring for me and helping me recover right from the beginning.

CHAPTER THREE

Recovery

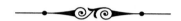

N ow the hard part began: Recovery.

Before this, I was rarely sick and didn't have much practice at letting people care for me. So the road to rehabilitation was challenging, right from the start.

There are two things I recall vividly during my stay in the hospital: my mouth being incredibly dry and Donna bringing me fresh pineapple slices and strawberries. Nothing had ever tasted so cool and refreshing. I also remember waking up after a long, deep sleep, wanting more fruit. Donna wasn't there and I panicked. I told the nurse in ICU I *had* to make an urgent call. It was 2 AM. Naturally, when Donna saw a call from University Hospital in the middle of the night, she thought I'd taken a turn for the worse. Poor thing. It was just me calling to ask for more pineapple.

I found it difficult to rely on others for my most basic needs, like getting food or going to the bathroom. I was not yet physically able to get up, but the idea of using that catheter just never sat well with me. I was miserable, and I wanted to go home. I begged the nurse to please let me go home, just for a while. I promised to return the next day. Since the nurse wouldn't cooperate, I took matters into my own hands. I bolted for the bathroom door, yanking out my IV and bleeding all over the place in the process. The nurse got me back in bed. As punishment (or for my own good, as my dad would say), I was strapped into the bed.

The next day I was off to the general ward. I didn't like it as well as ICU. The paging never stopped: "Clara Barton, to the nurse's stand." I heard it over and over again. I thought for sure she'd died right after the Civil War and was certainly not going to answer that page. To this day, I could swear that was the name I heard. Sounds get jumbled up in my head since the stroke. I can hear just fine, but I often hear something different than what was spoken to me.

I never lost my sense of humor throughout this ordeal. I often told Donna we had to either laugh or cry, and I preferred that we laugh.

More doctors came to examine me. They posed the same questions over and over. *What year is this? Who is the president?* The poor man in the next bed never did get those answers right, and you had to in order to go home. I felt bad for him.

A nurse came with medicine. Then there were more hospital folk poking and prodding me. (*No, I don't want some guy to give me a bath!*) Next came visits from a speech therapist and a physical therapist. It was exhausting and irritating. I just wanted to sleep and eat, like a baby. Now I understand that therapy must begin quickly so the brain cells that were shocked can recover. But at the time, it was just annoying.

In between hospital and therapy visits, I enjoyed seeing my family. My room was filled with flowers and cards. I felt the love, and it kept me going. No wonder Jesus gave us the great commandment to love. I witnessed its great power in my life, courtesy of family, friends and even strangers, when a nun stopped by to pray with me. At that time, my brain was functioning in many ways like a child's. So, I took everything literally. The nun said she was from Ireland. I remember thinking that was a long way to come to pray for me.

Through my entire ordeal, the constant love and comfort that I received kept me going. I never remember being afraid of death. That experience made me wonder more about this feeling we call *love*. I did some research and discovered that the Greeks had more than one word to describe love:

- Eros is the erotic love we experience with our sexual partners
- Philos is the brotherly love we have for our siblings
- Agape is unconditional love, like we have for our children

I believe that God's love is above all of these: a higher love that is more than we can comprehend during our time here on earth. It is a love so great that he will never abandon us, even when we sin and reject him. He makes the tough decisions for us, even when he must bear the pain of watching us suffer, in order to lead us to Heaven on earth and ultimately to his kingdom in Heaven above.

Days later, I answered all of the doctor's questions correctly, or maybe they just grew tired of me. I was released to a rehabilitation facility. This was not a pleasant experience for me. I was a spoiled executive accustomed to the comfort and service of a fine hotel when I was away from home. For some reason, I expected the same from rehab. I kept complaining to my wife that this was the Days Inn of rehab, and I wanted the Marriott.

She assured me that Walton was a first-class facility where I would be comfortable and get the rehabilitation I needed to go home. Donna was correct. At Walton I relearned many basic skills: walking; climbing and descending stairs; multitasking; and fine motor skills using my left hand. All of this was accomplished in only five days. I was a terrible patient (or the poster child for miraculous stroke recovery, as I prefer to remember it), and they released me to outpatient therapy.

God's love for me was evident. He put the right people in my life at the right time. This put me on the path to a full recovery and new discoveries on my life journey.

CHAPTER FOUR

Going Home

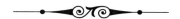

I will never forget my three-year-old granddaughter Maddie holding my hand, encouraging me and helping me maneuver the wheelchair. "You can do it, Pa. I'll help you." It's a natural reaction for an adult, but for Maddie it stemmed from just plain *love*. How blessed I was to have that little girl to cheer me on.

It was good to finally be back home. However, my life was dramatically different. Along with my physical disabilities, my voice and personality had changed. As a recent, involuntary member of the disabled stroke survivor group, I no longer possessed my signature quickness of mind. I learned what it was like to be part of an amazing, driven, hardworking group that no one joins by choice.

I remember being shocked the first time I was referred to as a "stroke survivor." It seemed silly. Was there any other option? I didn't recognize how close

I'd come to disaster. I now know that many don't survive the type of stroke I had. I was truly blessed.

Donna became my caregiver, which was difficult at first. Her daily prayer was, "Dear Lord, just give me something to work with." God answered her prayers.

I was lucky she took her job seriously, but that meant she pushed me hard each day. I was no longer her seemingly invincible husband. Gratefully, her training as a nursery school teacher benefitted both of us. She was a strict teacher, requiring that I got out of bed every day for therapy. (She rewarded me afterward with a trip to Arby's.)

She made my rehabilitation fun, by encouraging me to recite nursery rhymes. Those simple songs taught me how to vary the rate, pitch and volume of my speech, rather than using the new monotone voice I'd acquired after my stroke. I must admit, I changed some of the words to "Peter, Peter, Pumpkin Eater," but I can't repeat them here. It made us laugh instead of cry. I kept trying to find silly, new ways to make Donna laugh, because I knew she had a great burden to deal with during my recovery.

I never knew what day it was, so she made a chalkboard calendar to make it easier for me. One day, I told her that the chalkboard was nice, but it would be better if she also included the weather report, so I knew what to wear. She accommodated my request. We still laugh about that.

I was very forgetful early in my recovery. Often, I couldn't remember Donna's name, so every day I made up a new one. It went from "girl," to "ma'am," and my favorite, but the one she hated the most, "nurse." She got me back, though. The therapist suggested retraining my brain by throwing tennis balls to my left side, where I'd lost my peripheral vision. I don't think the therapist intended for her to throw so many balls quite so hard! When I complained, she'd say, "Doctor's orders!"

We continued to take one day at a time, but it was hard being six years old again. I was definitely a rebellious "child." Finally out of my infant stage, I rebelled against the strict caregiver Donna had become. I told her that I wanted my *sweet* wife back. She countered by reminding me, "I'm not the enemy!"

Like any child, everything that came into my mind came out of my mouth. It's never a good idea for a wife to know *everything* her husband is thinking. Especially when I saw a hot girl on television and asked her if I could have one. My adult filters were gone, and I had to find a way to regain them. Thankfully, I had a good and patient teacher.

I was in denial of my disabilities, right from the beginning. Still, thanks to my determination and Donna's tough love, I seemed to be on the way back to my normal life. Or so I thought.

My greatest triumph during that period was finding my way to the office of my speech therapist, Cindy, all by myself. I'd been going there for weeks, but each time she would come to the waiting room to lead me to her office. During a previous visit, Cindy taught me to develop a new skill to compensate for my disabilities. She helped me draw a map to her office. The visual made a big difference. Within a few visits I was able to find her office *without* the map. This is how I first learned to develop skills to compensate for my disabilities. The compensation skills Cindy taught me were critical components to my amazing recovery.

Tennis was a big part of my life before the stroke. It was fun, great exercise and a good way to make friends. Before the stroke, I never had a single tennis lesson. I was a natural athlete. Now, with my wounded body, I needed to learn how to play the game all over again. Oh, the patience Xavier the neighborhood tennis pro and my friends Pam and Trudy displayed on the tennis court. Thankfully, Xavier had worked with the disabled before. I was back on the court with Pam in no time; though she hit the ball directly to me every time.

It is truly a blessing to have good friends who accept you the way you are. I learned another important lesson about compensating for my disabilities. I could still play tennis, but I needed to resort to a different style of play. I was back on the court just two weeks after the stroke. My family and friends were stunned by my progress, but I was humiliated as I struggled to get my body and mind in sync.

But God's power is amazing. I am truly grateful that He showed his love for me by putting all the pieces of the puzzle together. He ensured that I encountered the right people, in the right place, at the right time. I believe God always answers our prayers; the Bible tells us so.

As I continued to go through my recovery, I had to shift my thinking. It was the toughest thing I've ever been through, but the outpouring of kindness from my family and community started to change my perspective of the world around me and my place in it.

When I got frustrated because I didn't get *immediate* answers to my prayers, I decided to be a little more open-minded about my journey. After all, what choice did I have? I could either become bitter or change my perspective.

Here is how I began to interpret God's answers to my prayers:

- Okay
- No, I have a better idea
- Not now

Perhaps the answer we receive isn't always the one we wanted. Still, it's usually the one that serves us best, even if we don't realize it in the moment. This is a lesson I would learn many times during the rest of my recovery, as I started a new phase of my life.

CHAPTER FIVE

Back to Work

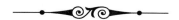

After months of rehab, keeping up with emails from home and learning how to drive again, I thought I was ready to go back to work. Work was a large part of how I defined myself before the stroke. Being a high-powered, corporate V.P. was my identity. Without it, a big piece of my life was missing. Physically, I felt fine, but I didn't realize how disabled my brain was.

In retrospect, I realize that I returned to work too soon to be successful in a demanding job, overseeing twenty-one drug stores. I wasn't the same person I was before the stroke. My employer wasn't able to accept me with my diminished capacities. I was inept at communicating. The subtleties of human communication, like sarcasm and innuendo, were lost on me. I often pleaded with Donna, "Just say what you mean."

My voice had also changed; I spoke softly. In meetings, when I tried to speak louder, it sounded aggressive. My store managers couldn't figure me out. They lost confidence in my ability to lead. I could see their frustration and feel their loyalties shift.

I struggled with my short-term memory and multitasking abilities. It was also difficult for me to stay focused and maintain energy throughout the day. Within a month, I was fired. This setback dealt a serious blow to my already wounded ego.

It was a bitter pill to swallow, but I had no choice. I went home and told my wife how angry and humiliated I felt. Frustrated by their decision, I blamed the whole thing on them. Didn't they know I had just come through one of the most trying times of my life?

I had been given so much love and support from my community. How could my employer, to whom I had devoted so much of my time,, show so little compassion? After much deliberation, we decided to accept their severance package, in lieu of any legal action, and move on with our lives.

I'd worked hard at rehabilitation to recover from the stroke and had come so far. I never considered failure an option. My experience as a high school athlete taught me to get back up, dust myself off and try again. My personal credo was: "You can knock me down, but you can't keep me down."

But with my mounting health issues and the betrayal of my company, it was just too much to bear.

I kept playing it over and over in my mind: If I couldn't go back to my prior job successfully, would I be able to get another job? Would I ever work again? What would I do if I couldn't work?

While I enjoyed time with family and friends, work always dominated my life. I could not accept a future without it. Physically, I felt fine, but I couldn't understand or accept my cognitive disabilities from the brain damage. So going on disability never occurred to me. Nor was it presented as an option by my employer.

CHAPTER SIX

What Now?

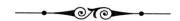

I'd tried going back to work and failed miserably. Never giving up hope or accepting my disabilities, I started a job search. Faced with an economic depression and having my age and my health working against me, I rarely got an interview. When I did, my cognitive disabilities worked against me, and I did not perform well.

Frustrated and desperate that no one would give me the dignity of a job, I decided to create my own. My childhood dream of owning a hardware store kept coming back to me. It seemed like the perfect time. I had the knowledge, the experience and the money to invest. My son and son-in-law wanted to join me. It would be wonderful working with family. I was convinced we could make it work. I invested all of our savings into opening a new hardware store in Myrtle Beach.

At that time, I was making decisions based heavily on emotions, rather than facts. I realized I was taking a risk, but I desperately wanted to work. Opening a family-owned hardware store felt like my best option. Unfortunately, this was the first of many poor decisions. We relied on what turned out to be bad information from a large hardware franchise. This led to a business plan that was doomed from the start. This ill-advised investment was compounded by a series of bad decisions that I made with my wounded business brain, like choosing this time to also build a new house.

We already owned a nice beach condo, free and clear, that we could have continued to live in until we established our new business. But I imagined having a big place for all the kids and grandkids to gather. This decision placed immediate pressure on our finances.

The pressure continued to mount, and soon Donna and I had no time for anything in our lives but work. Our loving relationship turned to that of "business partners," which led to bickering over many important decisions. This put a lot of stress on our marriage, and I found myself constantly frustrated. Just when we had built sales and cut expenses to a point where we could be profitable, along came the great recession of 2007.

Sales at the store took a nosedive and never recovered. As a result, we were evicted for failure to pay the rent five years after we'd opened the doors of our store. Still, we weren't ready to give up. We downsized and relocated the store. This bought us some time. We were able to hang on another two years before eventually finding ourselves in the same situation. It was depressing, and I was desperate for a solution.

Around this time, my daughter informed us that Yahoo! was looking for Americans who were struggling as a result of the tough economy to feature in their documentary reality series: *Remake America*. We certainly fit into that category, so we tried out for the show. We were selected to represent a mom and pop business. Our daughter Erin was selected to represent a single mom. Yahoo! paid us a small stipend and promised to provide resources to help us save our business. It was like a dream come true!

The extra money helped keep food on our table and gas in the cars. We were featured on the front page of Yahoo! News and gained worldwide publicity, which was followed closely by our local media. This resulted in publicity for the store and a few more customers. I was touched and surprised by how many strangers sent us money or product orders. Local residents even stopped by, offering their help. These were people like Jeff, our hardware angel, who did so much for us. He saw our story on Yahoo! and just showed up at our store one day, offering to work for free. He had spent a lifetime in the hardware business and we learned so much from him to help us improve the store. We are truly grateful for the blessings God showered upon us as a result of the Yahoo! documentary.

Our fifteen minutes of fame was exciting and seemed to help us turn things around. Then, suddenly, top management at Yahoo! changed, and the show was cancelled. It's amazing to me that to this day, people stop us on the street to say they followed the series and wondered how we were doing. Unfortunately, our newfound celebrity was too little and too late to save our store.

Then another spoiler: as sales finally reached a point where we could pay the bills, our landlord demanded all rent in arrears from all tenants. We'd just paid for the current month's rent, but were about a year behind. There was absolutely no way we could cough up $60,000 immediately. We found ourselves evicted again.

What a disappointment! At this point, I was really starting to lose faith in myself and even in God. Why was I going through all this hardship? What had I done to deserve failure after failure? Why wasn't I being rewarded for hard work and perseverance? I'd been asking for answers and was sure the hardware store was the solution. What was I missing?

I considered trying to find another landlord that would take a chance on me, but we had no capital for moving and startup expenses. Donna and I were exhausted. We'd been working seven days a week for years. We were both over sixty years old and we just didn't have the stamina for it.

Up to that point, our bank had still been backing us, but with no facility, they were forced to liquidate. I felt as if I was letting my family down as I watched our business circle the drain. I felt desperate to make it work. My value as a man and the breadwinner of my family was tied to being successful. At times, I let my pride get the better of me. I was angry and frustrated. The rollercoaster ride put additional strain on my marriage and family.

We needed to make a decision; it was time to stop the bleeding.

I'll never forget the last time Donna and I stopped by the store. The auctioneer had started to move some product around to prepare for the next day's auction. Donna's eyes teared up as she lamented, "My store, my beautiful store."

Goodbyes are always tough, especially for your children. The store felt like a child we'd nurtured since birth. From that point, I knew it was time to let go of the past and focus on the present to create a better future.

This got me thinking about a quote from Matthew: "Let today's problems be enough for today." I started focusing on living in the present. This later became one of my guiding principles for my H.OP.E. Philosophy, which I will address in greater detail later in the book. I knew I was in way over my head and I needed to turn to a higher power for guidance.

I remember thinking, "Only Almighty God can help us now."

We were in a desperate situation.

Our entire retirement savings was gone; all of it invested in our failed hardware store. We'd sold our beloved beach condo, where we'd spent so many memorable weekends, as collateral for the business. We lost it to foreclosure. All that remained was a small pension.

Donna and I subsisted on food that could be purchased at the dollar store. The bank had yet to foreclose on our primary residence, so we continued to live in our beautiful home, which we could no longer afford. It felt like homelessness was just around the corner.

Bill collectors were driving us crazy. We hated answering the phone. Donna had a recurring nightmare: a man would show up at the door, take everything and say, "This isn't enough, so I'll have to cut off your arm and take that, too."

Would our new normal be sleeping on my mother's couch back in Ohio? I'd already been turned down for disability once. I thought perhaps it was worth another try, as I could now show a path of trying to work for others, and myself, and failing.

It felt like I was in a freefall, hoping someone would catch me. I often considered Psalm 91 11:12 "For God commands the angels to guard you in all ways. With their hands they shall support you lest you strike your foot against a stone."

CHAPTER SEVEN

Looking for Someone to Catch Me

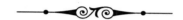

I t was a tremendously stressful period for us. Still struggling with my health issues, we now had to deal with our precarious financial situation, too. Overwhelmed, I searched for something to strengthen my faith and help me endure. I'd been raised Catholic, thanks to my dad, but unfortunately, I had yet to build my faith on a rock, as the Bible tells us.

I found Stasia's faith-sharing group through my local church, St. Andrew's Catholic Church. Faith sharing in small groups was a new concept for the congregation, and for me. It was structured as a way to help one another along life's challenging journey.

At this point, I felt like I was falling apart, unable to cope with all the blows life had dealt me. The first thing the group helped me with was becoming more aware of the daily *blessings* I encountered. This immediately provided a new, positive, central theme for my life.

Soon I began to see my glass as half full instead of half empty. I came to realize that my blessings far outnumbered my sorrows. I was blessed with a loving and devoted wife; children who supported and encouraged me; and grandchildren who looked up to their grandpa with unconditional love and devotion. This soon became the next phase of healing for me. I thanked God and the saints for my renewed faith.

In short, I learned to live in the present, rather than dwell on the past. I also came to realize there is more to life than working and making money. I listened intently while other group members shared their hardships. Some had lost a spouse or faced debilitating health problems. As a result, I realized that everyone faces hardships in life. I became more focused on praying for others, which helped lift the burden of my own problems.

I started to see my stroke as a second chance in life, an opportunity instead of a loss. The Hebrew phrase *La Heim*, meaning "To life!" is often used as a toast to health and wellbeing. Those words played repeatedly in my mind. They helped me to realize that I couldn't change reality, but I could change my perspective.

My daughters both bore twins around the same time, and I found myself wishing I had spent more time with my children when they were little. It all went by so fast, and I missed so much as I focused on moving up the corporate ladder. And for what? The wealth was all gone now.

As a grandpa, I could spend time with my grand-children and be involved with the things I missed with *my* kids, like school plays and birthday parties. What a blessing! Because of my stroke and my new per-spective, I felt like I was "living," perhaps for the first time...*La Heim*!

Reading the Bible and participating in group dis-cussions with my faith group became a new source of joy and inspiration for me. I looked forward to our weekly meetings and beyond the group for other learning opportunities. The more I learned, the hun-grier I became for more knowledge. Even though I struggled terribly from memory problems, somehow I was able to remember Scripture. Members of the faith sharing group expressed how much they enjoyed my reflections on the weekly readings. I credit this to God opening a window when a door closed. I had lost my executive-level brain function, but gained the ability to understand and explain Scripture to others.

Do you know how many people need this type of guidance in their lives? I felt truly blessed that God had called upon me to help others in this way.

I began thinking of the priest as a conduit through which Jesus spoke to me, to help me cope with my sit-uation. One of my favorite readings is a lesser-known story about Martha and Mary. Luke 10:38-42 tells of an occasion when Jesus was visiting with Martha and her sister, Mary. When he arrives Martha starts to worry and fuss about the visit. On the other hand, Mary simply falls at his feet and listens to Jesus.

Jesus says, "Martha, Martha, you are anxious and worried about many things. There is need of only one thing." Mary kept her eye on Jesus, listened to him and let the day unfold the way it was meant to. Sometimes I think I hear Jesus scolding me, as he did Martha. Then I stop worrying about all of the tasks on my "to do" list, and the problems of the day fade away.

The stories of Jesus, studied in the faith group, spoke to me. For instance, the story of how Jesus fed thousands with five loaves of bread and two fish (Matthew 14:13-17). When it was the end of the day, and the crowd grew hungry; Jesus said, "There is no need for them to go away; give them some food your-selves. The story continues in verse 19-21 where 'all ate and were satisfied" and had twelve wicker baskets of fragments left over.

This story taught me not to just sit back, do nothing and wait for God to bail me out of a bad sit-uation; but rather to take action, and Jesus would be right by my side. With faith I have the confidence to take action, and know it will work out.

I hired an attorney to appeal the disability rejec-tion. At first he was very discouraged about my sit-uation and hesitant to take the case. However, I was persistent, and he took me on as a client.

I learned to take life as it comes, *complete with the blessings that are often in disguise*. One of those blessings occurred by way of a new member who joined my faith group. He was a doctor, and I was in need of a new physician. As he assessed my health and my stroke recovery, he told me to forget about ever returning to my prior job. The brain damage was just too severe.

He recommended retiring on disability and assisted me in writing the necessary letters. As it so happened, one week prior to the store being closed by the landlord, I received a call stating that my disability payments had been approved and would start the following month.

What a gift from God! *Hallelujah!*

I decided to surrender completely to the will of God. I attended a retreat at another church, led by the singing priest Fr. James Diluzio. He taught me to think of my life as riding a bicycle built for two. God will steer, while I pedal. I don't need to worry about where we are going because I am armed with strength from the power and presence of God and life goes on, as it always does.

I had seen the goodness of God. He gave me the gift of disability payments when we were destitute. My prayers had been answered, but the question remained as to what I should do next in my life?

I kept applying and interviewing for jobs, but nothing worked out. I went back to the Scriptures for more guidance. I took a Bible study class on the Lord's Prayer and reflected on the complete meaning of this important lesson.

I believe that when Jesus spoke of everlasting life, he meant now and forever. The Lord's Prayer is loaded with instructions on how to live our lives and find hope. This prayer first names God, our Father. The Bible says to be childlike in our faith (Luke 18:16). In a simplistic way, I think this asks us to think of God as our (divine) Daddy, giving us direction as we interpret the Bible. Why should we complicate it any more than that?

This gives me the confidence I need to trust in his will for me, no matter what happens. It also assures me that he loves me unconditionally, like the love we receive from our earthly fathers and the love we have for our own children.

The prayer also teaches me to adore our God and Creator ("hallowed be thy name"), to give thanks and to accept his will ("thy will be done"). Even though it sounds simplistic in nature, focusing on our "daily bread" helps us stay in the present and be thankful for what we have today.

I also see that before the bread comes the wheat and before the wheat, the seeds. So I interpret this as instructing us to plant and cultivate what He gives us. We have the free will to decide whether or not to do this. He decides which seeds grow, according to His will for our lives.

The key for me is to listen carefully to God in meditation, so I know what seeds to plant and which to abandon. I pay close attention to all of the miniscule details in my life. I work hard, being sure to plant every good seed and till it carefully. Then I wait to see what grows.

For example, I heard God's call to join Stasia's group. After much perseverance, this eventually led me to accept my disabilities and the financial support from Social Security Disability Insurance. This put me on a path to harvest a much different life than I had planned, but in the long run, by letting go and letting God, it's been quite rewarding.

I discovered that His next plan for me was to help answer the prayers of another. But first, I had to learn how to listen for his voice. After Bible study one evening, I was driving home and noticed several new signs near the road which stated, "Food Pantry This Way."

I wondered if they were stocking the pantry and might need some help. God had just given me the gift of disability payments. So I was quite aware of what it felt like to fear where your next meal would come from. I drove past the pantry, thinking I would stop some other time. Then I heard a voice say, "You don't have to go to work anymore. Turn back!"

That was my first strong whisper from God.

I quickly turned around. Upon walking into the pantry, I was greeted by Wes and Shirley, who were in charge. I also met a young girl, about my daughter's age, named Veronica. Wes said she'd stopped by for food, but since the pantry wasn't well stocked, he'd been praying for someone to help her.

I gave Veronica ten dollars and she was thrilled that she'd be able to buy meat for her children. She explained that she lived with her sister, and that there were five children between them. Even though she had a job as a pharmacy tech at one of the drug store chains, her hours had been cut so severely she could no longer make ends meet.

She said she'd also driven past the signs, wondering if she should stop. Her pride was holding her back until she thought about how she'd put her twelve-year-old son to bed the night before with only a bowl of cereal to eat for dinner.

I remembered how I ate when I was twelve: a big dinner, plus seconds. Dad would laugh as I made a plate of ham sandwiches for my brothers and me to eat as a snack while we watched TV. I was grateful that God saw fit to use me to ensure Veronica and her son would have a meal that night.

Slowly but surely, I began to see little miracles unfold around me. I felt truly blessed when *I* could be the answer to someone else's prayer.

Veronica left to go to the grocery store and share the good news with her sister. Shirley, Wes and I had to celebrate this wondrous meeting and give thanks to God in Heaven.

Another example of God using me to answer the prayer of another occurred when we were forced to explore the possibility of bankruptcy as our debt from the hardware store spiraled.

I was in the attorney's office, about two weeks before Christmas, when a young woman and her little girl sat next to me. I love kids, so I asked the child what she wanted from Santa. She replied, "I want a purple dress."

I went on to my appointment with the lawyer, but the conversation with the little girl kept replaying in my mind. Thinking there was no way for her mother to purchase presents for her child, I mentioned the conversation to one of my employees. She immediately offered to purchase the purple dress. The next day I called the receptionist at the attorney's office, told her about the purple dress and asked her to put me in touch with the family. A few days later, we met the woman and her daughter, loaded with toys purchased with money that Donna and I scraped together, and of course, the purple dress.

I've come to realize that God has a plan for my life. In fact, He has a plan for all of us. Because of free will, we must search for it.

I am writing this today because in prayer I hear God calling me to do so. I keep wanting to go back to what is comfortable: working in retail. Yet, more and more, I realize I need to abandon the comfortable and find my destiny—the life I was meant to live since before creation. I believe God's plan for me; at this time is to write this story to inspire others, although that has been extremely difficult due to my disabilities. Typing is tedious. Life can be difficult at times. I think it is more of a boxing match than a knitting bee.

When I look for inspiration, I consider what the Apostle Paul said in his second letter to Timothy, at 2 Timothy 9, "He saved us and called us to a holy life, not according to our works but according to his own design and the grace bestowed on us in Christ Jesus before time began."

My previous pattern of living gave me short-term pleasure with the things money could buy. I now seek long-term joy that can be found through my spiritual connection. I regularly experience the same sentiment that King David expressed when he said of the Lord in Psalm 16:11, "You will show me the path to life, abounding joy in your presence."

My delight in life now comes from the heart to the brain, through the Holy Spirit. I appreciate the gift of another new day. I'm keenly aware of God's beautiful creation all around me. I focus on living like St. Joseph; I accept my situation and show love and tenderness to those who cross my path each day.

CHAPTER EIGHT

Charleston

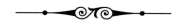

"There is never a dull moment, being married to you," Donna said, early one morning when we arose at my daughter's home in Charleston, eight years after my stroke.

We'd just moved to Charleston to spend more time with the grandchildren and lend support to our daughter. Erin was a single mom and the mother of twins. Our daughter had been struggling since her husband left. Erin was juggling the demands of work, managing finances and caring for two five-year-olds all by herself.

She definitely needed our support.

I had felt God calling me to Charleston for some time, but I was reluctant to just let go. Donna and I felt that the Myrtle Beach area was home. We were settled in, had lots of friends, new part-time jobs and our church. Then one day a recruiter from Publix supermarket called. I'd submitted my resume to them a few months before and had forgotten about it. The recruiter explained that they were expanding in the Carolinas and asked if I would be interested in Charleston with the opportunity to work my way back into management.

That was the nudge I needed, and God knew it so we moved to Charleston and rented a nice apartment. We are now in a position where we have plenty of good food and enough money to pay the bills and live comfortably. Our spirits are lifted each day by the smiles of our grandchildren.

God's plan has become clear. I had to learn that life wasn't just about work, and the power and money that gave me. It was about living life abundantly, with Jesus at my side.

The idea of starting over in the same place and manner as we had decades earlier—just the two of us, no money and an uncertain future—was thrilling. I was ready to begin our new life and never look back.

About a year after arriving in Charleston, I had the opportunity to return to work full time with one of the drug chains. The extra money would be nice, and I wanted to work again, while I had the opportunity. I now had the courage to try; knowing that I could trust in the goodness of God. My disabilities and age continued to work against me. It wasn't working out for either me or the drug chain so I thought it best to resign.

Since I was letting God steer me, I could not help but wonder why he led me down this path, when he knew I would fail. Since God's ways are not man's ways, I may never know; but I think it was all about healing my brain and body from the stroke. Donna could see continued improvement in my brain function when I returned to work. I have learned that stroke recovery will plateau. When that happens, I have to stretch myself, beyond my comfort zone by doing something new and challenging. It is really not any different than the process we go through growing up and moving past high school to college.

I also put on more than a few pounds when I slowed down after the stroke. I had been trying to drop 25 pounds, but was not able to do it. I really had to get my weight down, if I wanted a high quality old age. The combination of giving up sweets for lent, and going back to work, caused the pounds to fall off quickly. Yes, God understood what motivated me, so going back to work, was all about my health, not what I thought at all. I How could I serve him in the future,spreading the message of H.O.P.E. if I was in poor health?

Once again trusting in God, and letting the Holy Spirit guide me proved the best decision, even though, at times I wondered where we were going and why? Looking back, I now see the blessings in disguise, from yet another failure.I can now see God at work in my failures and my victories. It is nice to know that God will always be there to pick me up when I fall.

CHAPTER NINE

My Keys to H.O.P.E.

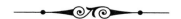

This book is simply my personal experience with a major, life-changing event, an account of how that helped me to more highly develop the spiritual side of my brain and a reflection on the relevance of drawing closer to God in today's society. The timelessness of the Bible is amazing to me. It is just as relevant today as it was when it was written over two thousand years ago. As I read scripture I ask myself four questions: 1) how does this make me feel? 2) What questions does it raise? 3) What does it teach me about God or life? 4) How will I apply it to my life?

Consider the words of John Chapter 1:

In the beginning was the Word
And the Word was with God.
And the Word was God
He was in the beginning with God

All things came to be through him
And without him, nothing came to be
What came to be through him was life
And this life was the light of the human race
The light shines in the darkness
And the darkness has not overcome it.

As I've mentioned, I lost many things: our homes, our wealth and my business acumen. (Donna says I am down with the normal people, like her, now). Along the way, a new, more spiritual part of my brain became activated. I believe that – if we choose to – we can experience **H**eaven **O**ur **P**romise on **E**arth (H.O.P.E.) by learning how to draw on this divine power.

Using this as a guiding light, I have broken down my journey into four personally proven steps that allow me to build on my faith and see miracles every day. I have listed them below with questions that may help you on your spiritual journey:

- **Holiness – Trust in your divine guidance, by living in a state of grace.** I learned how to do this through the Catholic Church, and my affiliation with my local faith group. Two powerful examples of the blessings I received as a result of trusting divine guidance include finding a new doctor and receiving disability insurance. *Q: Is there a safe place you can retreat to – in nature, with friends or perhaps a trusted organization – to find your spiritual connection?*

- **Others – Focus on the needs of others.** This was illustrated when I found the food pantry and realized how profoundly I could affect someone else's life. It happened again at the bankruptcy lawyer's office (of all places!) when I met the little girl who wanted a purple dress. *Q: How can you take action to help others in small, yet significant ways?*
- **Present – I can only find God in the present.** Living in the moment transforms into gratitude for simple things like having food on the table,, flowers in the garden, and the love of family and friends. *Q: Why worry about something in the future that may never happen?*
- **Evangelization – Read the Bible and spread the good news.** Help people shift the way they look at current circumstances that often become blessings (in disguise) when we look back later. If I have found silver linings after recovering from tragic situations, I'll bet you can too. *Q: Who could you uplift by sharing a Scripture that you personally find encouraging?*

Finding H.O.P.E. required me to first make a conscious decision to go "all in." Find a peaceful place to pray and *listen*. I prefer natural environments, like a garden, forest, or the beach. Looking at God's beautiful creations and soaking it all in helps me connect to my Creator by giving thanks.

I've found medical evidence to support this theory. According to Dr. Roizen and Dr. Oz in the *Post and*

Courier on 8/13/2013, "Getting up close and personal with Mother Nature yields big mind-body benefits." In the article, they outline how communing with nature strengthens our immunity, provides a break from worry and increases energy and creativity. For me, this is all part of the process of *finding Heaven on earth* as the Our Father Prayer teaches us. As Catholics we believe there are three persons, but one God. The Father is the creator, the Son the redeemer and the Holy Spirit the sanctifier.

The Holy Spirit lies deep within our soul. When I was struggling with going back to work, I prayed for guidance, and resigned from that job the next day. That was not the answer I was asking for, but eventually I realized it was the right path for me. When you let God steer you down *His* path, you may be in for a wild ride. I frequently pray to the Holy Spirit to send my guardian angels to help me. I heard that the Hebrew translation for Holy Spirit is "the wind", so I just trust that 'the wind will blow me in the right direction each day.

I also pray often to The Blessed Virgin Mary, our Holy Mother. These prayers usually are answered for me. I think it's hard for Jesus to say no to Mom.

In John Chapter Two, when the host of a wedding feast ran out of wine, Jesus turned water into wine to please his mother. The Memorare is a Catholic prayer to Mary that works for me when I'm desperate for help and feel as though I'm in a situation that only a higher power could handle. I also find peace when I am troubled by closing my eyes and visualizing that I am sending a spiritual bouquet of flowers to the Blessed Mother Mary. This prayer cured many a sleepless night when stress was at its highest point in my life. Both prayers can be found in the appendix of this book.

My daughter went through a bad financial crisis after her divorce. She was in danger of losing her home. I prayed passionately to the Blessed Mother Mary, asking for her intercession with her son Jesus, to save my daughter's home for the sake of her family. Sure enough, Erin got the loan modification on her mortgage. The most difficult, yet most important part of prayer, is listening to God's response

How do you do it? It requires getting still with your thoughts at certain times, yet also having the ability and openness of mind to pay close attention to everything happening around you. As a result, you may see little messages sent from on high.

I find that I must find a time when my mind is void of any thoughts, but at the same time open to "going with" any thought that God gives me. For me, that is when I am in a deep state of prayer, usually after Holy Communion (when I receive the body and blood of Jesus).or when meditating on my daily scripture readings

One day I was having difficulty living in the present, so I turned to my daily Bible reading for guidance. As I read Psalm 118, verse 24 kept coming back to me: "This is the day the LORD has made; let us rejoice in it and be glad." This is a good example of how God very subtlety answered my prayers for comfort that day. As a result, I let go of worry and handed my troubles over to God. This single mindset has helped me create a more peaceful way of living.

Sometimes I hear God connecting to me through songs on the radio, while driving. For me this is a time when my mind is free of any thought other than the boredom of driving the same old road ahead.. When the right song comes on it gives me guidance and lifts my spirits. I love this one:

"Have I told you lately that I love you? There is no one else above you." Knowing how much I am loved helps me feel confident as I put my trust in Him.

I believe Jesus wanted us to spread the good news of the gospel to bring Heaven to earth, and to prepare us for an eternity with Him in Heaven. The Catechism of the Catholic Church supports my conclusion when it says in paragraph 163, **"Faith-the beginning of eternal life**. Faith makes us taste in advance the light of the beatific vision, the goal of our journey here below. Then we shall see God 'face to face,' 'as he is.' So faith is already the beginning of eternal life."

The way I see it, Catholics believe God came to earth in the form of Jesus, so why wouldn't *He* want Heaven here as well?

Jesus (God, to me, the second person of the Holy Trinity, the Father, Son and Holy Spirit) promised salvation. There's no reason that shouldn't start now, as we learn to find H.O.P.E., the promise of Heaven on earth.

John 14:27 quotes Jesus as saying, "Peace I leave with you. My peace I give to you. Do not let your hearts be troubled or afraid."

CHAPTER TEN

In God's Hands

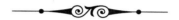

Thanks to God making the tough decisions for me, I can spend the balance of my time on body, mind and soul with a mix of work and leisure activities. I look forward to each day with the excitement of a child. I let the Holy Spirit guide me. I now have the faith to just enjoy the wild ride we call life.

I believe God lives a humble, anonymous existence. *As a result of what I've been through, I no longer fear death, and if I don't fear death, then why fear life?*

The Bible tells us 365 times not to be afraid. No accident that we were given one reminder for every day of the year.

The story of Peter walking on water, found at Matthew 14:22-33, taught me to keep my eye on Jesus and not be afraid. Peter was able to walk on water as long as he showed faith in Jesus. I can't walk on water, but I can live my life and trust that God knows what's best for me.

I believe that Heaven is not necessarily a place, but rather a state of being, where you live a balanced life completely in the present, without any worries. The following doctrine supports my conclusion.

Consider paragraph 2659 of The Catechism of the Catholic Church: "Time is in the Father's hands, it is in the present that we encounter him, not yesterday, nor tomorrow, but today." I know that with God, all things are possible (Mathew 19:26). To quote Jesus, in Mathew 11:28-30, "Come to me, all you who labor and are burdened, and I will give you rest. Take my yoke upon you and learn from me, for I am meek and humble of heart: and you will find rest for yourselves. For my yoke is easy, and my burden light."

CHAPTER ELEVEN

Final Thoughts and Conclusion

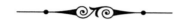

With this important shift comes a philosophy: Isn't living a heavenly life really about finding the silver lining in *everything?* The years since the stroke have been difficult, but my faith journey made me stronger. Consider this story from an unknown author, as applied to my story.

God came down from heaven to help me in my time of challenge. He told me to push on a big rock that was dropped in my yard.

Well, I pushed on that rock every day and prayed and prayed. Do you think I ever moved it even an inch? A year later, I complained to God that I did just what he told me, but I could not move that rock. God replied, "I never told you to move that rock. Don't you think if I wanted that rock moved, I could have done that myself with a snap of my fingers? Just look at how strong you got over the last year, pushing on that rock. I just wanted to make you stronger."

Pray
Until
Something
Happens

For years, I was trying to move that big rock (denying my disabilities) because I didn't want to see that life, as I knew it, was over. Now I'm thankful God intervened, moved the rock, and helped me grow into a spiritually stronger man with a new outlook on life.

Everyone has good and bad moods; however, since my stroke, I fight with severe depression that comes over me like a thick fog. I don't know what triggers it. I've tried prescription drugs and counseling; neither worked for me. Only the H.O.P.E. philosophy brings me out of it. I simply tell myself, "This is not Heaven on earth." Then I shift my outlook by going through each key to H.O.P.E. The relief comes from believing in God's plan, loving others, staying in the present and telling others my story.

Yesterday, for example, I asked myself: *When was the last time I prayed for someone else, or tried to make someone's day brighter in some small way?*

I hope this book has made your day a little brighter.

THE END (or is it?)

A Special Note From My Wife, Donna

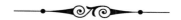

As Bill's wife, I went from a housewife to a caregiver in a few seconds. I became his coach, teacher and mom. We have been married for over 40 years. Through it all we have been best friends. I think that is one of the most important things to have in a marriage. We have lived all the vows: for better and worse, for richer and poorer, in sickness and in health, in good times and bad (I left out the obey part back then) and till death do us part.

In some ways, I have been married to two Bills (BS, before the stroke, and AS, after the stroke). We help take care of our grandchildren, and our part-time jobs give us a little fun money. We have made mistakes, but everything works out for the best. Bill has a tremendous faith and lately our prayers have been answered, so I keep telling him to think big. Winning the lottery would be nice.

Epilogue

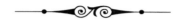

Without faith, there is no H.O.P.E. Consider this story from an unknown author, told to me by a priest in a homily:

Two frogs were sitting on a windowsill in a dairy farmer's kitchen. One frog had a strong faith in God; the other did not. Both frogs jumped off the sill and landed in a deep bowl of heavy cream.

They tried over and over to jump out, but the cream was too deep. They found themselves panicking, over their heads in trouble.

The frog with no faith simply said, "We are doomed." He gave up and drowned.

The other frog said, "I trust in God. I'm sure that he has a plan for my life, so I'm going to have faith." The faithful frog swam and swam. And prayed and prayed.

Sure enough, as he swam around the bowl, the cream turned into butter. Soon, all he had to do was jump on top of the butter, then jump again, out of the bowl.

This story helps me understand that God works in ways we don't always understand. We have to *trust*. I've seen this in my life when I've gotten in over my head. If I would have given up on God, I wouldn't have been open to accepting this dramatic change in the life I had planned. Now I appreciate the happiness of living in the present, not regretting past decisions orr worrying about the future.. I, trust that life will be good, wherever God leads me next. .I just keep on peddling, while God steers, and enjoy the wild ride.

APPENDIX

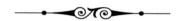

The following chapter includes Catholic prayers, and more information on Catholicism that were referenced in my prior text.

The Memorare

"Remember, Oh Most Gracious Virgin Mary, that never was it known that anyone who fled to your protection, implored your help, or sought your intercession was left unaided. Inspired by this confidence, I fly unto you, Oh Virgin of virgins, my mother; to you I come, before you I stand, sinful and sorrowful. Oh Mother of the Word Incarnate! Despise not my petitions, but in your mercy, hear and answer me. Amen.

Spiritual Bouquet to Mary the Blessed Mother (taught to me by Father Andy)

Send three spiritual rose bouquets to the Blessed Mother by reciting the Hail Mary prayer three times.

The first bouquet is white roses representing her goodness and purity, the second red to represent the sacrifice of her son. The third is gold representing the richness and happiness of my future.

'Hail Mary, full of grace.
The Lord is with thee.
Blessed are thou among women.
And blessed is the fruit of thy womb, Jesus.
Holy Mary, mother of God, pray for us, sinners, now and at the hour of our death.
Amen.

The Lord's Prayer (The "Our Father")

Our father, who art in heaven
Hallowed be thy name
Thy kingdom come, thy will be done
On earth, as it is in heaven
Give us this day our daily bread
And forgive us our trespasses
As we forgive those who trespass against us
Lead us not into temptation
But deliver us from evil
Amen.

The Great Commandment and the Ten Commandments

Love your God, with all your heart, all your soul, and all your mind. Love your neighbor as yourself.

1) I, the Lord am your God. You shall not have other gods besides me.
2) You shall not take the name of the Lord, your God in vain.
3) Remember to keep holy the Sabbath day.
4) Honor your father and your mother.
5) You shall not kill.
6) You shall not commit adultery.
7) You shall not steal.
8) You shall not bear false witness against your neighbor.
9) You shall not covet your neighbor's wife.
10) You shall not covet anything that belongs to your neighbor.

THE CATHOLIC FAITH

(The Apostles Creed)

I believe in God, the Father Almighty, Creator of Heaven and earth; and in Jesus Christ, His only Son, our Lord: Who was conceived by the Holy Spirit, born of the Virgin Mary; suffered under Pontius Pilate, was crucified, died and was buried. He descended into Hell; the third day He rose again from the dead; He ascended into Heaven, is seated at the right hand of God the Father Almighty; from thence He shall come to judge the living and the dead.

I believe in the Holy Spirit, the Holy Catholic Church, the communion of Saints, the forgiveness of sins, the resurrection of the body, and life everlasting. Amen.

Holy Communion (catechism #1331)

Holy Communion because by this sacrament we unite ourselves to Christ who makes us sharers in his Body and Blood to form a single body.

An Invitation to Learn More

The Catholic faith has given me the complete package for finding H.O.P.E. I was lucky to be raised Catholic. Anyone can join by completing the Rite of Christian Initiation of Adults (RCIA). Your local Catholic church can give you the details. More information on Catholicism is available at www.catholic.org

CPSIA information can be obtained
at www.ICGtesting.com
Printed in the USA
FFOW05n2350270415